Contents

Introduction

The Scarsdale diet is a very strict eating plan that allows for just 1,000 calories per day, regardless of your body size, sex, or activity level. No substitutions of any kind are allowed and each meal is specifically defined for each of the 14 days of the diet.

This is a high-protein program that also includes fruits and vegetables. You consume 43% of your calories from protein, 22.5% of calories from fat, and 34.5% of your calories from carbohydrates.

Dr. Tarnower is very explicit in his book that you are not to extend the program beyond 14 days. During the two weeks of the diet, he says that you will lose up to 20 pounds, which is unrealistically high and potentially unsafe.

After the 14-day weight loss phase, Dr. Tarnower outlines a lifetime "keep slim" plan. During this program, you follow a similar but slightly more relaxed version of the Scarsdale diet. For example, in the maintenance phase, you can have one alcoholic drink per day. The maintenance plan can be followed indefinitely, but if you start to gain weight (as defined as a four-pound weight increase on the scale), you are advised to go back on the 14-day Scarsdale diet.

Since the book has gone out of print, several websites are now dedicated to the program. These sites outline the 14-day meal plan and some provide recipes for the protein bread, a staple on the diet. But none of these sites are affiliated with the original program.

Chapter one

The diet's background and history

The Scarsdale diet started as a two-page diet sheet made by Tarnower to help his patients lose weight for better heart health.

After many individual success stories, Tarnower published the book "The Complete Scarsdale Medical Diet" in 1979.

The diet allows a mere 1,000 calories per day regardless of your age, weight, sex, or activity levels. It's heavy in protein, consisting of 43% protein, 22.5% fat, and 34.5% carbs.

The diet also forbids snacks and numerous healthy foods, such as potatoes, sweet potatoes, rice, avocados, beans, and lentils.

Tarnower died 1 year after the book's publication. Shortly thereafter, the Scarsdale diet was heavily criticized for its extreme restrictions and unrealistic weight loss promises. As such, the book is no longer in print.

How to follow the Scarsdale diet

The rules of the Scarsdale diet can be found in Tarnower's book "The Complete Scarsdale Medical Diet." Though it's no longer in print, some copies are still sold online, and some unofficial Scarsdale diet websites list its details.

The main rules include eating a protein-rich diet, restricting yourself to 1,000 calories per day, and following a limited list of approved foods. You are forbidden from any snacks except carrots, celery, and low sodium veggie soups, which are only to be eaten when necessary.

You must drink at least 4 cups (945 mL) of water per day but can also enjoy black coffee, plain tea, or diet soda.

Tarnower emphasized that the diet is only intended to last 14 days, after which you transition to the Keep Slim program.

Keep Slim program

After the 14-day initial diet, you're allowed to introduce a few banned foods, such as bread (up to 2 slices per day), baked goods (as a rare treat), and one alcoholic beverage per day.

While you're still expected to follow the list of approved foods, you're allowed to increase your portion sizes and calories to allow more flexibility.

Tarnower suggested following the Keep Slim program until you notice your weight increasing. If you regain weight, you're instructed to do the 14-day initial diet again.

What to Eat

- Limited vegetables
- Cheese and eggs
- Nuts
- Fruit (especially grapefruit)
- Meat, poultry, seafood, cold cuts
- Black coffee, tea, water, diet soda
- Protein bread

What Not to Eat

Butter, salad dressing, avocado, and most other fats

Potatoes, rice, sweet potatoes, beans

Sugar and sugary treats

Pasta, most bread, flour-based foods

Full fat milk

Alcoholic beverages

Limited Vegetables

Some vegetables, including leafy green vegetables, zucchini, green beans, and Brussels sprouts are usually part of the day's diet, generally at dinner. Carrots and celery are the only snacks allowed on the plan.

Cheese and Eggs

Eggs are included in a few lunch menus and can be prepared according to your preference as long as no fat is used. Cheese slices and cottage cheese are also included in a few lunch menus.

Nuts

Nuts are not included in the standard meal plan. However, on the substitute lunch plan, you are allowed to have six halves of walnuts or pecans.

Fruit

Grapefruit is included in every breakfast. It is also included in several lunches. Fruit salad is also included in a lunch menu.

Meat, Poultry, Seafood

Roast chicken and turkey, lamb, hamburger, and broiled steak are included in dinner menus. Fish and shellfish are also on a dinner menu. Cold cuts are included in lunch menus, although fatty meats such as bologna are not allowed.

Zero-Calorie Beverages

Black coffee, tea, water, and diet soda are included in the plan. Cream and sugar in your tea or coffee are not allowed.

Protein Bread

Protein bread (made with soy flour, whole wheat flour, and gluten flour) is a staple on this plan. A recipe is provided in the book, but this product was also available in grocery stores in the 1970s.

Alcoholic Beverages

No alcohol is allowed during the 14-day Scarsdale diet. However, on the maintenance plan, one serving is allowed per day.

Butter and Other Spreads

No added fat is allowed on the program, including butter, margarine, salad dressings, peanut butter, olive oil, or avocado.

Potatoes, Rice, Sweet potatoes, Beans

Starchy vegetables and legumes are not allowed on the plan as they are significant sources of carbohydrates.

Sugary Treats

No desserts of any kind (ice cream, baked goods, candy, etc.) are allowed on the program.

Pasta and Flour-Based Foods

No bread or pasta products ae consumed on the diet, except for specific amounts of protein bread.

Full Fat Milk

Only low-fat and nonfat milk products are allowed.

On the plan, you eat three meals per day. Snacks are not allowed, except for carrots and celery.

Pros and Cons

Pros

The rules are easy to follow, which makes this plan seem appealing. However, the drawbacks of the Scarsdale diet outweigh any potential benefits.

- Simple

The Scarsdale diet is easy to follow and leaves very little room for error. Each meal is outlined and includes only two to three foods. Substitutions are strongly discouraged. If you have a food allergy, substitutions are allowed, but otherwise, foods should be consumed exactly as indicated.

- Specific Meal Plan Provided

Consumers who don't like having to plan meals or count calories may prefer this program because it takes the guesswork out of meal planning. There is not a lot of variation from one meal to the next, so shopping should be simple and most foods (except for the protein bread) are easily found in most grocery stores.

- Inexpensive

Compared to weight loss programs that require you to buy prepackaged food, this program is likely to be less expensive. Food is consumed in very small quantities, so your grocery bill for the two weeks of the plan is not likely to be very high.

- No Subscription or Long-Term Commitment

Unlike many weight loss programs that are popular today, there is no subscription required to follow the Scarsdale diet. Consumers can simply buy the book (if they can find an available copy) or get one from the library to follow the plan.

Cons

Even for the 14 days it is designed to last, the Scarsdale diet is very restrictive, which could make it difficulty to follow and even unhealthy.

- Extremely Low in Calories

Everyone who follows the Scarsdale diet consumes 1,000 calories per day, regardless of age, sex, weight, or activity level. As a basis for comparison, most weight loss programs today set a calorie target of roughly 1,200–1,500 calories for women and 1,500-1,800 calories for men. Those who are very active generally consume more calories.

- Not Sustainable

While some people may be able to follow this program for two weeks, many people will find that the program is too restrictive to maintain. Researchers recommend that diets should be nutritionally adequate and tailored to meet individual needs in order to be sustainable for the long term.

- Limits Healthy Carbohydrates

During the two weeks that you follow the Scarsdale diet, your carbohydrate intake is substantially limited. While you will still consume healthy greens such as spinach and green beans, your intake of healthy fiber-rich foods like legumes and whole grains is severely restricted.

- Unrealistic Weight Expectations

A "desired weight chart" is provided in the book that readers can use as a guideline to see if they should lose weight. The chart does not take any factors other than sex into account. According to Dr. Tarnower, the chart is simply based on his years of medical experience.

By today's standards, the weight ranges Dr. Tarnower provided may seem restrictive. For example, the chart indicates that a 5' 4" woman should weigh between 110 and 123 pounds, which is on the lower end of the current healthy BMI recommendation.2 According to current recommendations, someone who is 5' 4" would fall between 110-145 pounds in order to have a BMI that falls within the "healthy" range.3 In addition, Dr. Tarnower's weight range offers no discussion of lean muscle mass or body composition.

Body Mass Index (BMI) is a dated, biased measure that doesn't account for several factors, such as body composition, ethnicity, race, gender, and age.

Despite being a flawed measure, BMI is widely used today in the medical community because it is an inexpensive and quick method for analyzing potential health status and outcomes.

The Scarsdale diet was widely compared to the Atkins diet when the program was first released. Both programs were developed by cardiologists in a medical setting and were provided to patients before being published in book form. But the Atkins program has changed substantially over the years and the programs are no longer comparable.

The Scarsdale diet does not adhere to the current recommendations provided by the USDA for protein, carbohydrate, or fat intake. According to the 2020–2025 Dietary Guidelines for Americans, adult men and women are advised to consume 10–35% of calories from protein, 45–65% of calories from carbohydrates, and 20–35% of calories from fat with an emphasis on healthy fats. The USDA also provides a recommendation for dietary fiber (approximately 22–34 grams per day).

On the Scarsdale diet, you consume 43% of your calories from protein, 22.5% of calories from fat, and 34.5% of your calories from carbohydrates. Fat intake comes primarily from saturated fat and fiber intake is low. The USDA recommends limiting your intake of saturated fats to less than 10% of daily calories.

Current dietary guidelines also suggest that calorie intake should be personalized and take into account a person's age, sex, weight, height, and level of physical activity. None of these factors are considered in the Scarsdale diet aside from an individual's sex. The calorie target provided for the duration of the two-week program is substantially lower than what current guidelines would suggest.

To lose weight, the USDA recommends a reduction of 500 calories a day. On a 2,000 calorie diet, that's an intake of roughly 1,500 calories a day, but this number, too, can vary.4 To get an estimate of your daily calorie needs, this calorie calculator takes into account personalized information to give you a healthy weight loss or weight maintenance goal.

Health Benefits

The Scarsdale diet restricts calories to create a calorie deficit, which will likely lead to weight loss. But any weight lost on this plan is likely going to be water weight. Current health recommendations advise that a safe and healthy rate of weight loss is 1 to 2 pounds per week.5 Anything more than that is typically unsustainable.

Health Risks

The very low-calorie intake and extreme weight loss promises of the Scarsdale diet have been heavily criticized by health experts. While current research on the Scarsdale diet is lacking since the official program is no longer available, a report from 1983 indicates that a woman was diagnosed with symptoms resembling porphyria, a rare blood disorder that is normally genetic, after following a three-week version of the Scarsdale diet.6

If calories and healthy carbohydrates are limited, it is possible that those following any iteration of this program will not meet the recommended daily allowance (RDA) for vital nutrients. For example, without whole grains or legumes, it would be challenging to meet the RDA for fiber. Research shows that low-carb, high-protein diets are notoriously low in fiber.7

Additionally, those who live active, healthy lifestyles may struggle to maintain their physical activity level on just 1,000 calories per day. You may feel lethargic, experience headaches, and have an overall decrease in motivation if you don't consume enough fuel each day. Highly restrictive diets may also not be appropriate for those who have had or are at risk for developing an eating disorder.

Sample 3-day menu

The Scarsdale diet recommends eating the same breakfast each day and drinking lukewarm water throughout the day. Snacks are banned, but you're allowed carrots, celery, or low sodium veggie soups if you can't wait until your next meal.

Furthermore, you aren't permitted to cook with oils or other fats and cannot add spreads to your protein bread.

Here's a 3-day sample menu for the Scarsdale diet:

Day 1

- Breakfast: 1 slice of protein bread (no spread), half of a grapefruit, and black coffee, tea, or diet soda
- Lunch: Salad (canned salmon, leafy greens, and vinegar and lemon dressing), plus fruit, as well as black coffee, tea, or diet soda
- Dinner: Roast chicken (no skin), spinach, half of a bell pepper, string beans, and black coffee, tea, or diet soda

Day 2

- Breakfast: 1 slice of protein bread (no spread), half of a grapefruit, and black coffee, tea, or diet soda
- Lunch: 2 eggs (no fat), 1 cup (162 grams) of low fat cottage cheese, 1 slice of protein bread

(no spread), plus fruit, as well as black coffee, tea, or diet soda

- Dinner: a lean hamburger (a large helping allowed), salad (tomatoes, cucumbers, and celery) with lemon and vinegar dressing, and black coffee, tea, or diet soda

Day 3

- Breakfast: 1 slice of protein bread (no spread), half of a grapefruit, and black coffee, tea, or diet soda
- Lunch: assorted meat slices, spinach (unlimited amounts), sliced tomatoes, and black coffee, tea, or diet soda
- Dinner: a grilled steak (all fat removed — a large serving allowed), Brussels sprouts, onions, half of a bell pepper, and black coffee, tea, or diet soda

Chapter two

Juicy Roasted Chicken

This roasted chicken is perfectly seasoned and just like the way my grandmother used to make it. The method used in this recipe results in the juiciest chicken! We loved to nibble on the celery after it was cooked.

Prep Time: 15 mins

Cook Time: 1 hr 15 mins

Additional Time: 30 mins

Total Time: 2 hrs

Servings: 6

Ingredients

1 (3 pound) whole chicken, giblets removed

salt and black pepper to taste

1 tablespoon onion powder, or to taste

½ cup butter

1 stalk celery, leaves removed

Directions

Preheat the oven to 350 degrees F (175 degrees C).

Place chicken in a roasting pan; season generously inside and out with onion powder, salt, and pepper. Place 3 tablespoons of butter in chicken cavity; arrange dollops of remaining butter on the outside of chicken. Cut celery into 3 or 4 pieces; place in the chicken cavity.

Bake chicken uncovered in the preheated oven until no longer pink at the bone and the juices run clear, about 1 hour and 15 minutes. An instant-read thermometer inserted into the thickest part of the thigh, near the bone, should read 165 degrees F (74 degrees C).

Remove from the oven and baste with drippings. Cover with aluminum foil and allow to rest for about 30 minutes before serving.

Nutrition Facts (per serving)

423 Calories 32g Fat 1g Carbs 31g Protein

Perfect Roast Chicken

Want a roasted chicken that is juicy inside without the use of a baking bag or flour? Then this recipe is perfect. It is quick and easy to prepare. The picture shown does display a chicken that was cooked in a bag, but the chicken was also roasted with vegetables and needed the bag to immerse the vegetables in the chicken flavor. I still guarantee a juicy chicken without the use of a bag each and every time.

Prep Time: 15 mins

Cook Time: 2 hrs

Total Time: 2 hrs 15 mins

Servings: 6

Yield: 1 whole roasted chicken

Ingredients

1 (4 pound) whole chicken

1 cup margarine, softened

1 tablespoon garlic salt

1 teaspoon coarsely ground black pepper

1 teaspoon dried thyme

1 teaspoon dried parsley

1 pinch dried rosemary

Directions

Preheat oven to 350 degrees F (175 degrees C).

Rinse and pat chicken thoroughly dry with paper towels. Mix margarine, garlic salt, black pepper, thyme, parsley, and rosemary in a bowl and rub the outside of the chicken thoroughly with the margarine mixture. Place any remaining margarine mixture into the cavity of the chicken. Place chicken into a glass baking dish.

Bake chicken in the preheated oven until browned and the juices run clear, about 2 hours. An instant-read meat thermometer inserted into the thickest part of a thigh, not touching bone, should read at least 160 degrees F (70 degrees C).

Nutrition Facts (per serving)

650 Calories 53g Fat 1g Carbs 41g Protein

Happy Roast Chicken

The easiest and best roast chicken recipe! I use organic chickens.

Prep Time: 5 mins

Cook Time: 1 hr 15 mins

Additional Time: 15 mins

Total Time: 1 hr 35 mins

Servings: 4

Yield: 1 roast chicken

Ingredients

½ cup dry white wine

2 lemons, cut in half

6 large cloves garlic

1 (4 pound) whole chicken

1 ½ teaspoons cold butter

2 tablespoons Dijon mustard

salt and pepper to taste

Directions

Preheat an oven to 425 degrees F (220 degrees C). Pour the wine into a 10-inch cast-iron skillet; set aside.

Place the lemon halves and garlic cloves into the cavity of the chicken. Slide half of the butter underneath the skin of each breast. Rub the chicken all over with Dijon mustard, then season to taste with salt and pepper. Place into the cast-iron skillet.

Bake the chicken in the preheated oven for 15 minutes, then reduce heat to 350 degrees F (175 degrees C), and continue baking until no longer pink at the bone and the juices run clear, about 1 hour more. An instant-read thermometer inserted into the thickest part of the thigh, near the bone should read 180 degrees F (82 degrees C). Remove the chicken from the oven, cover with a doubled sheet of aluminum foil, and allow to rest in a warm area for 15 minutes before slicing.

Nutrition Facts (per serving)

638 Calories 36g Fat 11g Carbs 62g Protein

Roast Chicken with Rosemary

This rosemary roasted chicken is inspired by my time in Italy. When I was in Vicenza at a downtown open-air market, I smelled scrumptious roast chicken from a stand. So, I bought one and saw what they stuffed in the cavity to make it taste so good. I prepare turkey this way, too.

Prep Time: 10 mins

Cook Time: 2 hrs

Total Time: 2 hrs 10 mins

Servings: 6

Ingredients

1 (3 pound) whole chicken, rinsed

salt and pepper to taste

1 small onion, quartered

¼ cup chopped fresh rosemary

Directions

Preheat the oven to 350 degrees F (175 degrees C).

Season chicken all over with salt and pepper, including cavity. Stuff cavity with onion and rosemary. Place chicken in a 9x13-inch baking dish or roasting pan.

Roast in the preheated oven until chicken is no longer pink in the center and the juices run clear, 2 to 2 1/2 hours. An instant-read thermometer inserted into the center of chicken near the bone should read at least 165 degrees F (74 degrees C).

Recipe Tip

The cook time will vary depending on the size of your chicken.

Nutrition Facts (per serving)

291 Calories 17g Fat 1g Carbs 31g Protein

Caribbean-Spiced Roast Chicken

Tropical flavors make this chicken really delicious.

Prep Time: 15 mins

Cook Time: 1 hr 30 mins

Total Time: 1 hr 45 mins

Servings: 4

Yield: 1 chicken

Ingredients

1 ½ tablespoons fresh lime juice

2 fluid ounces rum

1 tablespoon brown sugar

¼ teaspoon cayenne pepper

¼ teaspoon ground clove

½ teaspoon ground cinnamon

½ teaspoon ground ginger

1 teaspoon black pepper

½ teaspoon salt

½ teaspoon dried thyme leaves

1 (3 pound) whole chicken

1 tablespoon vegetable oil

Directions

Preheat oven to 325 degrees F (165 degrees C).

In a small bowl, combine the lime juice, rum, and brown sugar; set sauce aside.

Mix together the cayenne pepper, clove, cinnamon, ginger, pepper, salt, and thyme leaves. Brush the chicken with oil, then coat with the spice mixture.

Place in a roasting pan, and bake about 90 minutes, until the juices run clear or until a meat thermometer inserted in thickest part of the thigh reaches 180 degrees F. Baste the chicken with the reserved sauce every 20 minutes while it's cooking. Allow chicken to rest for 10 minutes before carving.

Nutrition Facts (per serving)

508 Calories 29g Fat 5g Carbs 46g Protein

Hard-Boiled Egg Sandwich

These are so good! I have been making these hard-boiled egg sandwiches for years and we absolutely LOVE them. This is a great on-the-go breakfast or just a different way to use up leftover hard-boiled eggs. Enjoy!

Total: 10 mins

Prep: 10 mins

Servings: 1

Yield: 1 sandwich

Ingredients

2 slices white bread, toasted

1 tablespoon butter, softened

2 tablespoons whipped cream cheese

1 hard-boiled egg, sliced

5 dashes hot pepper sauce (such as Frank's RedHot®), or to taste

1 pinch salt and ground black pepper to taste

Directions

Butter each slice of toast. Spread 1 tablespoon cream cheese onto each slice.

Layer hard-boiled egg slices evenly onto 1 slice of toast. Add hot sauce, salt, and pepper. Top with other slice of toast.

Substitute your favorite bread for the white bread, if you prefer.

Nutrition Facts

Per Serving: 372 calories; protein 11.2g; carbohydrates 26.9g; fat 24.4g; cholesterol 262.2mg; sodium 860mg.

Hard-Boiled Egg Casserole

Delicious and filling egg casserole which uses an unusual main ingredient: hard-boiled eggs! This is a much requested favorite for game-day brunch during football season.

Cook: 30 mins

Total: 45 mins

Prep: 15 mins

Servings: 8

Yield: 8 servings

Ingredients

8 hard-boiled eggs, peeled and halved

¼ cup butter

¼ cup all-purpose flour

2 cups half-and-half

½ teaspoon salt

¼ teaspoon ground black pepper

¼ teaspoon garlic powder

¼ teaspoon dry mustard

1 cup shredded Gruyere cheese

½ cup freshly grated Parmesan cheese

Directions

Preheat oven to 350 degrees F (175 degrees C). Butter a 9-inch square baking dish.

Arrange eggs, cut-side down, in the prepared baking dish.

Melt butter in a saucepan over medium-low heat. Whisk flour into the melted butter until dissolved, 2 to 3 minutes. Gradually stir half-and-half into flour mixture until sauce is thickened and smooth, about 5 minutes. Season sauce with salt, pepper, garlic powder, and mustard. Stir Gruyere cheese into sauce until melted and smooth.

Pour sauce over eggs and sprinkle Parmesan cheese over sauce.

Bake in the preheated oven until bubbling and golden brown, 20 to 25 minutes.

Nutrition Facts

Per Serving: 300 calories; protein 14.5g; carbohydrates 6.5g; fat 23.9g; cholesterol 268.9mg; sodium 395mg.

If you don't like the dry yolks and rubbery whites in traditional hard-boiled eggs, try making them using your sous vide immersion cooker. The yolks come out super moist and tender and never discolored, which makes the added cook time well worth the wait! Use any number of eggs; the directions remain the same.

Cook: 40 mins

Total: 45 mins

Prep: 5 mins

Servings: 6

Yield: 6 eggs

Ingredients

6 large eggs

Directions

Fill a large pot with water and place a sous vide immersion cooker into the water. Set temperature to 170 degrees F (77 degrees C) according to manufacturer's instructions. Once water is up to temp, slowly lower eggs into the water using a slotted spoon. Set timer for 40 minutes

Remove eggs from water once timer is up and place in a large bowl. Slowly shake bowl around to gently crack the eggs. Cover with ice water to cool. Peel carefully under running water.

Cook's Note:

The fresher the eggs, the harder they are to peel, so I like to use eggs that are a few weeks old for best results.

Nutrition Facts

Per Serving: 72 calories; protein 6.3g; carbohydrates 0.4g; fat 5g; cholesterol 186mg; sodium 70mg.

How to Make Perfect Hard Boiled Eggs

This method makes the most perfect hard-boiled eggs ever. The whites are firm but not rubbery, and the yolks are cooked and still creamy.

Cook: 5 mins

Additional: 40 mins

Total: 50 mins

Prep: 5 mins

Servings: 6

Yield: 6 hard-boiled eggs

Ingredients

6 eggs

Directions

Place eggs into a saucepan and pour in cold water to cover; place over high heat. When the water just starts to simmer, turn off heat, cover pan with a lid, and let stand for 17 minutes. Don't peek.

Pour out the hot water and pour cold water over eggs. Drain and refill with cold water; let stand until eggs are cool, about 20 minutes. Peel eggs under running water.

Nutrition Facts

Per Serving: 72 calories; protein 6.3g; carbohydrates 0.4g; fat 5g; cholesterol 186mg; sodium 70mg.

Soft Hard-Boiled Eggs

Here's my foolproof method for making hard-boiled eggs when we want softer, creamier yolks such as in salads. The steaming method is very precise, so you may need to experiment with different times, depending on the size of the eggs and the temperature of your fridge.

Cook: 9 mins

Total: 12 mins

Prep: 3 mins

Servings: 6

Yield: 6 servings

Ingredients

1 ¼ cups water

6 large cold eggs

Directions

Place water into a 3-quart saucepan with a lid. Place over high heat and bring to a low boil. Carefully place the eggs in the water. Cover pan immediately, reduce heat to medium-high, and cook for 9 1/2 minutes. Remove pan from heat and cool eggs down with cold running water, tipping out the water, and continuing to run cold water over the eggs until they are cool.

Cook's Note:

The steaming method is very precise, so you may need to experiment with different times, depending on the size of the eggs and the temperature of your fridge.

If you gently crack the shells of the cooked eggs during the rinsing/cool down step, the water seeps in between the shell and egg and makes them extremely easy to peel.

Nutrition Facts

Per Serving: 72 calories; protein 6.3g; carbohydrates 0.4g; fat 5g; cholesterol 186mg; sodium 71.5mg.

Soft-Boiled Eggs in the Microwave

After reading numerous articles on the subject of soft-boiled eggs, I came up with a recipe that gave consistent results that you will enjoy.

Cook: 5 mins

Total: 10 mins

Prep: 5 mins

Servings: 2

Yield: 2 eggs

Ingredients

water

2 eggs

½ teaspoon salt

Directions

Fill a bowl with warm water and place cold eggs into the bowl, to keep from cracking when you cook them.

Fill a microwave-safe bowl with water; add salt. Microwave on high power to boil, 1 to 1 1/2 minutes.

Place warm eggs into the bowl of hot water and cover the bowl with plastic wrap.

Place the bowl of covered eggs into the microwave and microwave on 60% power for 1 1/2 minutes.

Remove from the microwave and transfer eggs to a bowl of cool water to stop the cooking process. Peel and serve.

Cook's Note:

Cook times may vary some, depending on what microwave is used.

Nutrition Facts

Per Serving: 72 calories; protein 6.3g; carbohydrates 0.4g; fat 5g; cholesterol 186mg; sodium 654.9mg.

Easy Hard-Boiled Eggs

I've tried many different ways to make a great, easy, hard-boiled egg with a soft white and a nice fluffy yolk that's not grey on the outside. After lots of trial and error, I've finally done it. After cooking I usually keep them in the shell until I need them. Enjoy!

Cook: 10 mins

Additional: 20 mins

Total: 35 mins

Prep: 5 mins

Servings: 6

Yield: 6 eggs

Ingredients

6 eggs

Directions

Place eggs into a saucepan and fill with water until eggs are just barely covered.

Bring water to a boil. Boil eggs for 4 1/2 minutes. Remove from heat and let eggs sit in hot water for 20 minutes.

Transfer eggs to a bowl and either peel and serve, or keep shells on and place in the refrigerator until you are ready to serve.

Nutrition Facts

Per Serving: 72 calories; protein 6.3g; carbohydrates 0.4g; fat 5g; cholesterol 186mg; sodium 70mg.

Try this never-fail method of cooking hard-boiled eggs for a dozen eggs that are perfect for snacking, using in salads, or making deviled eggs.

Cook: 20 mins

Additional: 15 mins

Total: 40 mins

Prep: 5 mins

Servings: 12

Yield: 12 eggs

Ingredients

water, as needed

12 eggs, at room temperature

12 cubes ice cubes

Directions

Fill a pot with enough water to cover all eggs. Bring to a boil. Lower eggs gently into the boiling water using a slotted spoon.

Return to a gentle boil and cook for 13 to 15 minutes, depending on how firm you want the yolks. Remove from heat and drain water, keeping eggs in the pot.

Fill the pot quickly with cold water to cool eggs. Add ice to speed the process.

When eggs are cool enough to handle, remove each one and gently crack the shell on all sides, without removing any shell. Place eggs back in the cold water and let stand for 15 minutes. Peel and remove egg shells to serve.

Nutrition Facts

Per Serving: 63 calories; protein 5.5g; carbohydrates 0.3g; fat 4.4g; cholesterol 163.7mg; sodium 62.8mg.

Perfect Hard-Boiled Eggs

I believe this to be the perfect recipe for hard-boiled eggs. The eggs peel so easily, most can be peeled in one simple motion. The egg yolk itself is a nice yellow color without the greenish tinge that sometimes occurs when making hard-boiled eggs.

Cook: 5 mins

Additional: 25 mins

Total: 35 mins

Prep: 5 mins

Servings: 12

Yield: 12 eggs

Ingredients

12 eggs

Directions

Fill a large pot halfway with water, making sure the pot is large enough to contain eggs in a single layer. Bring to a boil over high heat.

Place eggs in boiling water individually using a large spoon, making sure not to break them. Continue to boil for 1 minute. Remove from heat, cover, and let stand for 25 minutes.

Place eggs under cold water until eggs have cooled.

Cook's Note:

Water should be filled between 3 to 4 inches above eggs.

Nutrition Facts

Per Serving: 63 calories; protein 5.5g; carbohydrates 0.3g; fat 4.4g; cholesterol 163.7mg; sodium 61.6mg.

Creamy Cottage Cheese Scrambled Eggs

Cottage cheese eggs for breakfast are a nice change from regular scrambled eggs. This egg recipe comes out creamy and soft. Perfect with a slice of tomato and turkey bacon for a delicious and fast low-carb breakfast.

Prep Time: 5 mins

Cook Time: 5 mins

Total Time: 10 mins

Servings: 2

Ingredients

1 tablespoon butter

4 large eggs, beaten

¼ cup cottage cheese

1 teaspoon chopped fresh chives, or to taste (Optional)

ground black pepper to taste

Directions

Gather all ingredients.

Melt butter in a skillet over medium heat. Pour beaten eggs into the skillet; let cook undisturbed until the bottom of the eggs begins to firm, 1 to 2 minutes.

Stir cottage cheese and chives into eggs and season with black pepper.

Cook and stir until eggs are nearly set, 3 to 4 minutes more.

Nutrition Facts (per serving)

224 Calories 17g Fat 2g Carbs 6g Protein

Cinnamon-Peach Cottage Cheese Pancakes

A cottage cheese-based pancake with fruit for extra flavor.

Prep Time: 10 mins

Cook Time: 30 mins

Total Time: 40 mins

Servings: 4

Yield: 12 pancakes

Ingredients

4 eggs

1 cup cottage cheese

½ cup milk

1 teaspoon vanilla extract

2 tablespoons butter, melted

1 peach, shredded

1 cup all-purpose flour

2 tablespoons white sugar

1 pinch salt

¾ teaspoon baking soda

1 teaspoon ground cinnamon

Directions

Mix eggs, cottage cheese, milk, vanilla, butter, and peach in a large bowl. Combine flour, sugar, salt, baking soda, and cinnamon in a small bowl. Stir flour mixture into the cottage cheese mixture until just combined.

Heat a lightly oiled griddle over medium-high heat. Drop batter by large spoonfuls onto the griddle, and cook until bubbles form and the edges are dry. Flip, and cook until browned on the other side. Repeat with remaining batter.

Nutrition Facts (per serving)

344 Calories 14g Fat 36g Carbs 18g Protein

Cottage Cheese Chicken Enchiladas

Ever tried chicken enchiladas made with cottage cheese? Now's your chance! This takes some prep time, but it is well worth it. You can make it 1 day ahead, and serve the next day.

Prep Time: 30 mins

Cook Time: 30 mins

Total Time: 1 hr

Servings: 6

Yield: 6 servings

Ingredients

1 tablespoon vegetable oil

2 skinless, boneless chicken breast halves - boiled and shredded

½ cup chopped onion

1 (7 ounce) can chopped green chile peppers

1 (1 ounce) package taco seasoning mix

½ cup sour cream

2 cups cottage cheese

1 teaspoon salt

1 pinch ground black pepper

12 (6 inch) corn tortillas

2 cups shredded Monterey Jack cheese

1 (10 ounce) can red enchilada sauce

Directions

To Make Meat Mixture: Heat oil in medium skillet over medium high heat. Add chicken, onion and green chile peppers and saute until browned, then add taco seasoning and prepare meat mixture according to package directions.

To Make Cheese Mixture: In a medium bowl mix sour cream with cottage cheese and season with salt and pepper; stir until well blended.

Preheat oven to 350 degrees F (175 degrees C).

To Assemble Enchiladas: Heat tortillas until soft. In each tortilla place a spoonful of meat mixture, a spoonful of cheese mixture and a bit of shredded cheese. Roll tortillas and place in a lightly greased 9x13 inch baking dish. Top with any remaining meat and cheese mixture, enchilada sauce and remaining shredded cheese.

Bake at 350 degrees F (175 degrees C) for 30 minutes or until cheese is melted and bubbly.

Nutrition Facts (per serving)

549 Calories 31g Fat 34g Carbs 33g Protein

This cottage cheese egg bake is the easiest and best casserole I have tried so far. My sweet mother-in-law shared this recipe with me. I make 3 or 4 at a time and keep them in the freezer to take to gatherings, feed guests, or surprise kids. Green chiles make it pop!

Prep Time: 15 mins

Cook Time: 45 mins

Total Time: 1 hr

Servings: 10

Yield: 1 (10x13-inch) casserole

Ingredients

cooking spray

2 (16 ounce) packages cottage cheese

10 large eggs, beaten

1 pound shredded Monterey Jack cheese

1 (4 ounce) can diced green chiles

½ cup butter, melted (Optional)

½ cup all-purpose flour

½ cup cooked crumbled bacon (Optional)

1 teaspoon baking powder

Directions

Preheat the oven to 400 degrees F (200 degrees C). Grease a 10x13-inch baking dish with cooking spray.

Mix together cottage cheese, beaten eggs, Monterey Jack cheese, green chiles, melted butter, flour, bacon, and baking powder in a large bowl until well combined; pour into the prepared baking dish.

Bake in the preheated oven for 15 minutes. Reduce heat to 350 degrees F (175 degrees C) and continue baking until a toothpick inserted into the center of casserole comes out clean, about 30 minutes more.

Recipe Tips

You can use low-fat, low-moisture shredded mozzarella and skip the butter and meat for a healthier version. It tastes just as amazing!

You can use turkey bacon or Canadian ham instead of bacon if desired.

The casserole can be made the night before and refrigerated or frozen for later.

Nutrition Facts (per serving)

277 Calories 19g Fat 7g Carbs 19g Protein

Cottage cheese, fresh green onions, cucumbers, and tomatoes make this cottage cheese salad recipe great with spaghetti or other Italian favorites!

Prep Time: 10 mins

Total Time: 10 mins

Servings: 4

Ingredients

1 (16 ounce) container cottage cheese, drained

4 roma (plum) tomatoes, chopped

4 green onions, chopped

2 medium cucumbers, peeled and diced

salt and pepper, to taste

Directions

In a medium bowl, stir together cottage cheese, tomatoes, green onions, and cucumbers. Season with salt and pepper to taste. Chill until serving.

Nutrition Facts (per serving)

138 Calories

5g Fat

8g Carbs

15g Protein

Polish Noodles (Cottage Cheese and Noodles)

This simple recipe for pasta with cottage cheese came from the Polish side of my family. We call it "cottage cheese and noodles" or "lazy man pierogies." It's a great comfort food and can be made with any kind of noodle. You can serve it as a side dish, but we always enjoy it as a main course.

Prep Time: 5 mins

Cook Time: 15 mins

Total Time: 20 mins

Servings: 8

Ingredients

½ cup butter

1 small onion, diced

1 (16 ounce) package egg noodles

1 (16 ounce) container cottage cheese

½ cup sour cream

½ teaspoon sea salt

¼ teaspoon ground black pepper

Directions

Melt butter in a saucepan over medium heat. Cook and stir onion in melted butter until softened, 7 to 10 minutes.

Meanwhile, bring a large pot of lightly salted water to a boil. Add egg noodles and cook, stirring occasionally, until partially cooked, about 5 minutes. Drain and return to the pot.

Pour onion mixture over noodles, then stir in cottage cheese, sour cream, salt, and pepper. Cook over medium heat, stirring occasionally, until sauce is heated through and noodles are tender, yet firm to the bite, 5 to 8 minutes.

Nutrition Facts (per serving)

409 Calories 20g Fat 43g Carbs 16g Protein

Cottage Cheese Bread

This cottage cheese white bread is a hearty recipe I put in my bread machine — the kids just love it. I have also used nonfat cottage cheese.

Prep Time: 5 mins

Cook Time: 3 hrs

Total Time: 3 hrs 5 mins

Servings: 12

Yield: 1 1/2-pound loaf

Ingredients

½ cup water

1 cup cottage cheese

2 tablespoons margarine

1 egg

1 tablespoon white sugar

¼ teaspoon baking soda

1 teaspoon salt

3 cups bread flour

2 ½ teaspoons active dry yeast

Directions

Add ingredients to your bread machine in the order suggested by the manufacturer, and start. You can use up to 1/2 cup more bread flour if dough seems too sticky.

Nutrition Facts (per serving)

171 Calories 4g Fat 27g Carbs 7g Protein

Ribeye steak, seasoned salt, and pepper are all you need for a perfectly grilled steak. Make sure your briquettes are red hot.

Prep Time: 5 mins

Cook Time: 6 mins

Rest Time: 4 mins

Total Time: 15 mins

Servings: 1

Can You Double or Triple This Charcoal-Grilled Steak Recipe?

Of course! This recipe serves one, but it's easy to adjust the ingredients to feed two people or even a crowd. As long as you use one teaspoon of seasoned salt and one teaspoon of cracked black pepper per steak, the recipe should turn out perfectly.

Ingredients

1 (12 ounce) ribeye steak

1/2 teaspoon seasoned salt, such as Lawry's® Seasoned Salt

1/4 teaspoon freshly cracked black pepper, or to taste

Directions

Gather the ingredients.

Season steak evenly, using 1/4 teaspoon seasoned salt and 1/8 teaspoon black pepper on each side. Set aside.

Light charcoal briquettes. Once they are red hot, place steak on the grates. Grill for 4 to 5 minutes. Turn steak over and grill an additional 2 to 3 minutes.

Tent steak with aluminum foil and let rest 4 to 5 minutes before serving.

Nutrition Facts (per serving)

924 Calories 65g Fat 1g Carbs 85g Protein

Caprese Salad with Grilled Flank Steak

This is a fresh, healthy, easy-to-make salad with a twist to the usual restaurant versions. It can be served in large portions as a main course or in smaller portions as an appetizer salad.

Prep Time: 20 mins

Cook Time: 10 mins

Additional Time: 5 mins

Total Time: 35 mins

Servings: 4

Yield: 4 main course salads

Ingredients

2 medium tomatoes, diced

1 (4 ounce) ball fresh mozzarella, cut into 1-inch cubes

¼ cup coarsely chopped fresh basil

2 cloves garlic, minced, divided

41 tablespoons olive oil, divided

1 pound flank steak

salt and ground black pepper to taste

1 (6.5 ounce) bag butter lettuce mix

2 tablespoons balsamic vinegar, or to taste

Directions

Mix tomatoes, mozzarella, basil, 1 clove minced garlic, and 1 tablespoon olive oil in a bowl; toss to coat. Cover bowl and refrigerate.

Preheat an outdoor grill for medium-high heat and lightly oil the grate.

Place steak in a large resealable bag; add 1 clove minced garlic, 1 tablespoon olive oil, salt, and pepper. Seal the bag and distribute the oil mixture over the steak.

When the grill is preheated, cook steak to your desired degree of doneness, about 5 minutes per side for medium. An instant-read thermometer inserted into the center should read 140 degrees F (60 degrees C). Let stand for 5 minutes before thinly slicing across the grain.

Divide lettuce onto 4 serving plates. Drizzle 1 1/2 teaspoons each balsamic vinegar and olive oil onto each lettuce portion. Divide steak and tomato mixture evenly between the salads.

Nutrition Facts (per serving)

321 Calories 24g Fat 6g Carbs 20g Protein

Grilled Steak Salad with Sesame Dressing

Grilled steak salad with a sesame-rice vinegar dressing.

Prep Time: 30 mins

Cook Time: 15 mins

Additional Time: 1 hr

Total Time: 1 hr 45 mins

Servings: 2

Ingredients

1 (12 ounce) rib eye steak

1 tablespoon soy sauce

1 teaspoon Montreal steak seasoning, or to taste

½ lemon, juiced

2 tablespoons rice vinegar

2 tablespoons olive oil

2 tablespoons white sugar

½ teaspoon sesame oil

¼ teaspoon garlic powder

2 pinches red pepper flakes

10 leaves romaine lettuce, torn into bite-size pieces

½ large English cucumber, cubed

1 avocado - peeled, pitted, and diced

1 tomato, cut into wedges

1 carrot, grated

4 thin slices red onion

3 tablespoons toasted sesame seeds

Directions

Season both sides of rib-eye steak with soy sauce and steak seasoning. Cover and refrigerate at least 1 hour to overnight.

Preheat an outdoor grill for medium-high heat and lightly oil the grate.

Grill steak on preheated grill until firm, reddish-pink, and juicy in the center, about 6 minutes per side. An instant-read thermometer inserted into the center should read 130 degrees F (54 degrees C). Transfer steak to a platter, sprinkle with lemon juice, and cover loosely with aluminum foil. Allow meat to rest for about 10 minutes, then cut into strips.

Whisk rice vinegar, olive oil, sugar, sesame oil, garlic powder, and red pepper flakes together in a small bowl. Combine lettuce, cucumber, avocado, tomato, carrot, red onion, and steak strips in a large bowl. Pour rice vinegar dressing over salad and toss to coat. Sprinkle with sesame seeds to serve.

Nutrition Facts (per serving)

704 Calories 53g Fat 39g Carbs 26g Protein

This grilled flat iron steak is something I made for a Valentine's Day dinner. It turned out delicious! The flavored butter is what makes this dish.

Prep Time: 15 mins

Cook Time: 10 mins

Additional Time: 45 mins

Total Time: 1 hr 10 mins

Servings: 4

Ingredients

2 tablespoons red wine vinegar

2 cloves garlic, minced

1 tablespoon cracked black pepper

1 teaspoon dried rosemary leaves, crumbled

1 teaspoon dried oregano

¼ teaspoon kosher salt

¼ cup olive oil

1 ½ pounds flat iron steak

3 tablespoons softened unsalted butter

1 ounce crumbled blue cheese

1 tablespoon chopped fresh chives

⅛ teaspoon cracked black pepper

Directions

Whisk olive oil, vinegar, garlic, 1 tablespoon black pepper, rosemary, oregano, and kosher salt together in a bowl and pour into a resealable plastic bag. Add steak, coat with the marinade, squeeze out excess air, and seal the bag. Marinate in the refrigerator for 30 minutes.

Preheat an outdoor grill for medium-high heat and lightly oil grate. Remove steak from the marinade, shake off excess, and discard remaining marinade. Allow steak to stand at room temperature as the grill warms.

Meanwhile, mash butter, blue cheese, chives, and 1/8 teaspoon of black pepper together until combined; set aside.

Cook steaks on the preheated grill until firm and reddish-pink and juicy in the center, about 5 minutes per side. An instant-read thermometer inserted into the center should read 130 degrees F (54 degrees C). Allow steak to rest in a warm place for 10 minutes before slicing thinly across the grain. Serve with a dollop of blue cheese-chive butter.

Nutrition Facts (per serving)

551 Calories

44g Fat

3g Carbs

37g Protein

Steak Dry Rub Seasoning

This amazing steak seasoning is made with smoked paprika, oregano, garlic, and cumin. Rub onto any cut of steak and let sit for 15 to 20 minutes before grilling. Any extra dry rub can be stored in an airtight container for later use.

Prep Time: 5 mins

Total Time: 5 mins

Servings: 6

Yield: 1 cup

How to Store Steak Seasoning

Store steak seasoning in an airtight container in a cool, dry place (like your pantry). It should remain fresh for six months — but you can check that it's still good by giving it a quick sniff. If it doesn't smell like anything, it's time to toss it.

Ingredients

3 tablespoons kosher salt

3 tablespoons smoked paprika

2 tablespoons onion powder

2 tablespoons garlic powder

2 tablespoons dried oregano

2 tablespoons coarsely ground black pepper

1 tablespoon light brown sugar

1 tablespoon ground cumin

Directions

Gather all ingredients.

Mix kosher salt, smoked paprika, onion powder, garlic powder, oregano, black pepper, brown sugar, and cumin together in a sealable container. Seal container and shake to mix.

Season steaks.

Editor's Note:

The magazine version of this recipe uses 2 tablespoons of kosher salt.

Nutrition Facts (per serving)

49 Calories 1g Fat 11g Carbs 2g Protein

Skillet-Braised Brussels Sprouts

Braised Brussels sprouts are a quick and easy side dish for any meal. After being quickly sauteed in bacon grease, the Brussels sprouts are skillet-braised in chicken stock until tender then finished with a buttery balsamic and bacon pan sauce.

Prep Time: 10 mins

Cook Time: 15 mins

Total Time: 25 mins

Servings: 4

Ingredients

4 slices thick-cut bacon, sliced into 1/4-inch strips, or more to taste

1 pound Brussels sprouts, trimmed and halved lengthwise

1 clove garlic, thinly sliced, or more to taste

½ cup chicken stock

1 tablespoon butter, or to taste

1 tablespoon balsamic vinegar, or to taste

salt and ground black pepper to taste

Directions

Cook bacon in a large cast iron skillet over medium heat until just crisp, 5 to 7 minutes. Transfer to a paper towel-lined plate, reserving bacon grease in the skillet.

Place Brussels sprouts in the skillet with the cut-sides down. Increase heat to medium-high and saute in the bacon grease until lightly browned, 2 to 3 minutes.

Add garlic and saute until fragrant, about 30 seconds.

Pour in chicken stock and cover skillet with a lid; simmer until Brussels sprouts are bright green, 3 to 5 minutes. Remove the lid and continue simmering, until liquid is evaporated and sprouts are at desired tenderness, 3 to 5 more minutes.

Remove skillet from the heat. Add bacon, butter, balsamic vinegar, salt, and pepper; stir until butter is melted.

Recipe Tips

Use a skillet large enough to cook Brussels sprouts in a single layer. This will enable them to brown more evenly.

If you like your sprouts softer, add a little more stock and braise them for longer.

Nutrition Facts (per serving)

207 Calories 16g Fat 11g Carbs 7g Protein

These roasted Brussels sprouts taste sweet and salty at the same time. They're really good and very easy to make. The sprouts should be brown with deliciously crispy bits on the outside when done.

Prep Time: 15 mins

Cook Time: 30 mins

Total Time: 45 mins

Servings: 6

How to Roast Brussels Sprouts In the Oven

Here's a brief overview of what you can expect when you roast Brussels sprouts at home:

Place the ingredients in a zip-top bag and shake to coat.

Transfer to a baking sheet.

Bake until very dark brown, shaking often to promote even cooking.

Can You Roast Frozen Brussels Sprouts?

No fresh produce on hand? No problem. Prepare frozen Brussels sprouts exactly as you would in the standard recipe. Toss in oil, seasonings, and bake to a lovely seared, fork-tender finish. There's no need to thaw, saving you valuable time in the kitchen.

Ingredients

1 ½ pounds Brussels sprouts, ends trimmed and yellow leaves removed

3 tablespoons olive oil

1 teaspoon kosher salt

½ teaspoon freshly ground black pepper

Directions

Gather all ingredients.

Preheat oven to 400 degrees F (205 degrees C).

Place trimmed Brussels sprouts, olive oil, kosher salt, and pepper in a large resealable plastic bag. Seal tightly, and shake to coat.

Pour onto a baking sheet, and place on center oven rack.

Roast in the preheated oven for 30 to 45 minutes, shaking pan every 5 to 7 minutes for even browning. Reduce heat when necessary to prevent burning. Brussels sprouts should be darkest brown, almost black, when done. Adjust seasoning with kosher salt, if necessary. Serve immediately.

Serve hot and enjoy!

Recipe Tip

Any leftovers can be reheated or even just eaten cold from the fridge.

Nutrition Facts (per serving)

104 Calories

7g Fat

10g Carbs

3g Protein

Brussels Sprouts Gratin

A great way to have Brussels sprouts with a little more flair. The cream takes away the bitterness you usually find in Brussels. This is a family favorite during the holidays!

Prep Time: 15 mins

Cook Time: 35 mins

Additional Time: 10 mins

Total Time: 1 hr

Servings: 4

Yield: 4 servings

Ingredients

1 pound Brussels sprouts, cleaned and trimmed

2 slices bacon, cut into 1/2 inch pieces

salt and ground black pepper to taste

½ cup heavy cream

¼ cup bread crumbs

¼ cup grated Parmesan cheese

2 tablespoons butter, cut into tiny pieces

Directions

Preheat an oven to 400 degrees F (200 degrees C). Lightly grease a baking dish.

Bring a large pot of lightly salted water to a boil. Add the Brussels sprouts and cook uncovered until tender, about 8 minutes. Drain in a colander, then immediately immerse in ice water for several minutes until cold to stop the cooking process. Once the Brussels sprouts are cold, drain well, and cut in halves or quarters, depending on size. Set aside.

Meanwhile, place the bacon in a large, deep skillet, and cook over medium-high heat, turning occasionally, until limp and lightly browned, about 5 minutes. Reduce heat and stir in the Brussels sprouts. Season with salt and pepper then toss for about 1 minutes to evenly distribute the seasonings. Arrange bacon and Brussels sprouts on the prepared baking dish. Pour cream evenly over the Brussels sprouts, then sprinkle breadcrumbs and Parmesan cheese on top. Distribute pieces of butter over the bread crumbs.

Bake in the preheated oven until golden brown and heated through, 20 to 25 minutes.

Nutrition Facts (per serving)

312 Calories 25g Fat 16g Carbs 8g Protein

Garlic Brussels Sprouts with Crispy Bacon

Pan-fry Brussels sprouts in butter and crispy bacon for a smoky addition to your vegetable side dish. You can add a little of the bacon grease to the dish if you prefer.

Prep Time: 15 mins

Cook Time: 25 mins

Total Time: 40 mins

Servings: 6

Yield: 6 servings

Ingredients

1 ½ pounds fresh Brussels sprouts

8 slices bacon

1 teaspoon butter

2 teaspoons olive oil

4 cloves garlic, chopped

½ cup reduced-sodium chicken broth

¼ teaspoon salt

⅛ teaspoon ground black pepper

2 teaspoons butter

Directions

Cut an 'X' in the core end of each Brussels sprout. Set sprouts aside.

Place bacon in a large skillet and cook over medium-high heat, turning occasionally, until evenly browned, about 10 minutes; drain and cool on paper towels. Crumble.

Heat 1 teaspoon butter and olive oil in a large skillet over medium heat; cook and stir garlic until golden brown, 3 to 5 minutes. Add Brussels sprouts; toss to coat. Stir in broth, salt, and black pepper; cover and cook until Brussels sprouts are tender, 12 to 14 minutes. Drain liquid from pan.

Stir remaining 2 teaspoons butter into Brussels sprouts mixture until melted. Mix in bacon and serve.

Nutrition Facts (per serving)

151 Calories 9g Fat 11g Carbs 9g Protein

Conclusion

The Scarsdale diet gained widespread popularity because the substantial weight-loss claims it made were appealing to many people. While this specific diet is no longer popular, many other weight loss programs that make similar claims are widely promoted.

It's important to critically evaluate any claims made by a diet program or nutritional plan that you choose to undergo. In general, a healthy rate of weight loss is 1 to 2 pounds per week. Programs that promise much more than that may use methods that don't promote good nutrition or wellness. When in doubt, talk to your healthcare provider or speak to a registered dietitian to get personalized advice.

Remember, following a long-term or short-term diet may not be necessary for you and many diets out there simply don't work, especially long-term. While we do not endorse fad diet trends or unsustainable weight loss methods, we present the facts so you can make an informed decision that works best for your nutritional needs, genetic blueprint, budget, and goals.

If your goal is weight loss, remember that losing weight isn't necessarily the same as being your healthiest self, and there are many other ways to pursue health. Exercise, sleep, and other lifestyle factors also play a major role in your overall health. The best diet is always the one that is balanced and fits your lifestyle.